YOUR KNOWLEDGE HAS VALUE

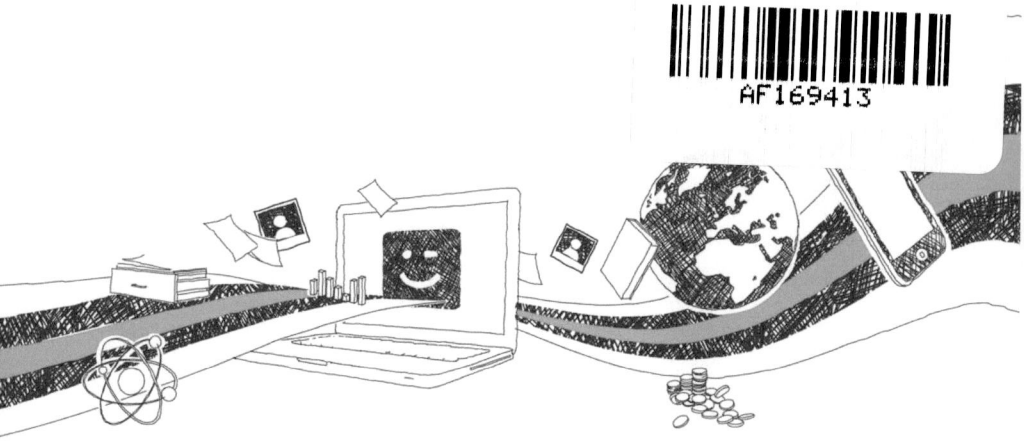

- We will publish your bachelor's and master's thesis, essays and papers

- Your own eBook and book - sold worldwide in all relevant shops

- Earn money with each sale

Upload your text at www.GRIN.com
and publish for free

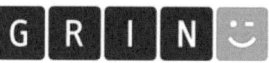

Bibliographic information published by the German National Library:

The German National Library lists this publication in the National Bibliography; detailed bibliographic data are available on the Internet at http://dnb.dnb.de .

This book is copyright material and must not be copied, reproduced, transferred, distributed, leased, licensed or publicly performed or used in any way except as specifically permitted in writing by the publishers, as allowed under the terms and conditions under which it was purchased or as strictly permitted by applicable copyright law. Any unauthorized distribution or use of this text may be a direct infringement of the author s and publisher s rights and those responsible may be liable in law accordingly.

Imprint:

Copyright © 2018 GRIN Verlag
Print and binding: Books on Demand GmbH, Norderstedt Germany
ISBN: 9783668626904

This book at GRIN:

https://www.grin.com/document/388293

Patrick Kimuyu

Malaria. Uganda's Progress in Achieving Millennium Development Goal #6C Target

GRIN - Your knowledge has value

Since its foundation in 1998, GRIN has specialized in publishing academic texts by students, college teachers and other academics as e-book and printed book. The website www.grin.com is an ideal platform for presenting term papers, final papers, scientific essays, dissertations and specialist books.

Visit us on the internet:

http://www.grin.com/

http://www.facebook.com/grincom

http://www.twitter.com/grin_com

Malaria: Uganda's Progress in Achieving Millennium Development Goal #6C Target

Name: Patrick Kimuyu

In theory, epidemiological transitions are enhanced by designing of appropriate health strategies aimed at achieving sustainability in the global healthcare system. Therefore, approaches towards the achievement of universal access to healthcare by the global population will reduce mortality rates and improve health in general. This is the core approach adopted by the World Health Organization through the implementation of MDG #5: improving maternal health, MDG #4: reducing child mortality and MDG #6 combating malaria and other infectious diseases. It has been reported that various countries around the globe have recorded diverse progress towards achieving the principal MDG targets, especially with regard to MDG #6. However, the achievement of MDG 6; target 6C depends on the commitment of different countries. It is worth noting that, some countries have recorded remarkable progress towards the reversal of malaria incidence rate while others have lagged behind owing to historical, cultural, structural and critical factors. For instance, Uganda is among the countries which have recorded remarkable progress towards the achievement of MDG 6C target, although it has not met other target objectives of MDG #6. Therefore, this argumentative paper will provide a comprehensive evaluation of Uganda's progress in combating malaria, and provide appropriate recommendations.

Ideally, a comprehensive critical analysis on Uganda's progress towards the achievement of MDG #6C target can be presented through providing an overview on the current situation in the country. The history of malaria in Uganda encompass an array of aspects owing to the fact that the country lies within the tropical region where malaria is known to be endemic. In regard to the country profile, Uganda is positioned between latitudes 4^0 North and 1^0 South of Equator. On the other hand, the country lies in a high altitude of 1,300-1,500M above the sea level (Mallinga et al., 2009). As such, Uganda experiences tropical climatic conditions owing to its geographical location. Ordinarily, the country experiences varied temperatures depending on the country's geography in which temperatures range from 16^0C in the Southwest to 30^0C in the Northeastern region (Adams & Spielberg, 2011). As a result, the country is covered with savannah woodland, tropical rain forests and semi-desert conditions, and these climatic conditions influence epidemiological trends of malaria, in which some regions experience more or less malaria prevalence rates than others.

In regard to the structure of Uganda's healthcare system, the formal healthcare system comprises of private for-profit sector, private not-for-profit sector and the public sector. Epidemiological surveys indicate that Uganda's public healthcare sector consists of referral hospitals which serve an approximation of 2 million people, and parish-level healthcare centers serving about 5,000 people. In addition, there are community health centers within the country's public healthcare sectors which are responsible for providing healthcare services to patients at the community level. As such, community health centers provide mobile healthcare services in collaboration with community medicine contributors (CMDs) and village health teams. Ordinarily, these parish-level healthcare centers and referral hospitals provide curative and preventive healthcare services to patients (Mallinga et al., 2009). However, it is worth noting that, Uganda has an extensive informal healthcare sector that contributes significantly in addressing healthcare challenges including combating malaria in the country.

Despite the remarkable advances realized by the Uganda's healthcare system in combating malaria transmission, malaria has been found to be one of the most challenging diseases in the country because it causes significant mortality, morbidity and economic loss. According to epidemiological data, malaria causes its greatest impact on children less than five years of age and pregnant women. This is attributable to biological factors related to the immune levels among children and pregnant women. In Uganda, malaria has been found to be causing 9-14 percent of the total inpatient deaths (Ahaibwe & Kasirye, 2012). On the other hand, malaria has been found to be responsible for 15-20 percent of hospital admissions, and it accounts for 30-50 percent of hospital visits (Acton, 2013). This implies that, malaria causes the highest percentage of the disease burden in the country's healthcare system. Currently, Uganda has been ranked 6th in the list of the countries with the highest incidence rates for malaria.

In addition, it has been ranked 3rd among the leading countries with the highest malaria deaths, and this implies that, Uganda experiences enormous consequences from malaria transmission. In reality, malaria transmission in Uganda ranges from 90-95 percent, although transmission is influenced by epidemiological variations in which over 320 malaria related deaths occur daily (Kagolo, 2013). In theory, areas of malaria transmission in Uganda can be divided into three principal epidemiological zones depending on the level of transmission. According to epidemiological surveys, 70 percent of the country comprises of high transmission levels in which infective bites per person exceeds 100, annually. The second epidemiological zone comprises of medium to high transmission levels in which 10-100 infective bites occur annually, accounting for 20 percent of total malaria transmission in the country. On the other hand, low transmission areas in which infective bites are less than 10 bites per person accounts for 10 percent. These are regarded to as stable perennial malaria transmission areas. There are also areas with unstable malaria transmission in which incidence rates of malaria are relatively low, especially in the Southwest region of the country that comprises of mountain ranges with altitudes of above 1,800 meters.

From an analytical perspective, Uganda seems to have realized a remarkable progress towards the achievement of MDG #6C target because epidemiological surveys show a significant reduction of malaria cases. Beaudrap et al (2011) reaffirm "malaria is a major public health problem, especially for children, however, recent reports suggest a decline in the malaria burden" (p. 132). In practice, the rate of Uganda's progress in combating malaria can be explained through a comprehensive evaluation of mortality rates of the populations that are at a high risk of malaria. Therefore, mortality rates of children under the age of 5 years can be used as the principal indicator of malaria reduction in Uganda. According to a recent epidemiological report from UNICEF (2013), child mortality related to malaria has been decreasing in the past two decades, and this is attributable to changes of health policy in Uganda. In this period, malaria related mortality rates among children aged less than five years seem to have decreased by 75 percent from 178, in 1990 to 69, in 2012. On the other hand, annual rate of malaria related mortality rates reduction indicates that, 2000-2012 accounted for the highest mortality reduction rates in the history of Uganda. In this period, Uganda recorded a reduction rate of 6.3% compared to the rates recorded in 1990-2000 and 1970-1990 periods corresponding to 1.9% and 0.1%, respectively.

Malaria Under-5 Mortality Rates

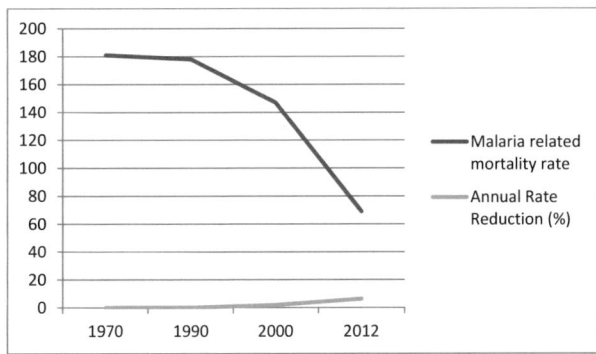

Source: UNICEF (2013)

In general, malaria related mortality rates exhibit similar trends in all other population groups including pregnant women, and this considered as a remarkable progress towards combating malaria in Uganda (Jensen, 2009).

From an epidemiological perspective, MDG #6C has been found to have immense impacts on patients, families, communities and the Ugandan government. Chimp Corp (2013) reports "management of malaria has a lot of implications ranging from individual, family to national levels. About 15 percent of premature death is due to malaria; most families spend close to 25 percent of their income on malaria treatment contributing to high levels of poverty in most households" (par. 7). Therefore, Uganda's progress in combating malaria has reduced the burden experienced by patients and families, al large. For instance, families are no long incurring enormous financial losses that used to be caused by malaria because its transmission has been reduced through the adoption of appropriate health policies, primarily malaria policy. This aspect can be evidenced by the reduction of the population below the poverty line, which was found to have reduced to 38% by 2011. This was far much below the percentage recorded in 1990 because the Ugandan population experienced adverse impact from the burden of malaria compared to the reduced burden at present.

Another significant influence of Uganda's progress towards achieving MDG #6C is the increase of life expectancy of the Ugandan population in which life expectancy increased from 47.5, in 1990 to 58 in 2012 (UNICEF, 2013). This implies that, morbidity related to malaria transmission has declined drastically in the past decade.

In theory, the progress realized by Uganda in combating malaria has been facilitated by the country's health policy approaches, including malaria policy that encompasses an array of objectives. Zaramba (2010) reports "the goal of malaria control in Uganda is to control and prevent malaria morbidity and mortality, minimize social effects and economic losses attributable to malaria in the country" (p. 26).

Uganda's malaria policy has led to the improvement of healthcare facilities and the establishment of appropriate malaria intervention and control approaches. Some of these approaches that have led to the reduction of malaria transmission include vector control through the use of indoor residual spraying, use of long-lasting insecticide treated nets, prevention of malaria infection during pregnancy and treatment. In addition, Uganda has been able to respond to malaria epidemics through the establishment of a reliable disease surveillance system that involves early detection and monitoring of drug resistance by malaria vectors in all epidemiological zones (Memoire, 2011).

Despite the progress realized by Uganda in reducing malaria transmission, there are several challenges faced by the country that seem to hinder the achievement of MDG #6C by 2015 (Kansiime, 2013). Some of these changes are cultural beliefs, illiteracy among the Ugandan population, access to universal healthcare services and cultural lifestyle.

Cultural beliefs appear to be one of the challenging issues related to the reduction of malaria transmission in Uganda. This is so because; a significant percentage of the Ugandan population does not pay attention to conventional medicine; instead, most people depend on traditional medicines as the mainstay for treatment. This implies that, treatment outcomes are compromised by the absence of disease diagnosis procedures to confirm malaria infection (Acton, 2012). On the other hand, malaria symptoms such as fever are similar to other health conditions; thus, traditional medicine experts confuse malaria symptoms with other diseases such as colds leading to wrong treatment. This aspect increases mortality risk because untreated malaria may cause death in the long run.

On the other hand, literacy level in Uganda has been found to be low, especially among women. Ordinarily, malaria prevention and control approaches aim at increasing people's understanding on treatment options. Therefore, women who are concerned with caring for neonatal babies lack adequate education that can enable them to predict malaria in their children. This situation is complicated by the lack of universal healthcare services, in which malaria patients including children fail to receive treatment during the early stages of infection.

Moreover, cultural practices such as nomadic lifestyle in which some communities move from one area of the country to another with their livestock create difficulties in providing malaria treatment to them. It is difficult to establish health facilities in areas inhabited by nomadic communities because they do not stay in these areas permanently.

In a brief conclusion, Uganda has realized remarkable progress in combating malaria. This is attributable to its health policy that has proven reliable for implementing malaria prevention and control strategies. Despite these challenges, Uganda appears to be advancing progressively towards achieving MDG #6C. Its success in reducing malaria related mortality by more than half in the past 10 years is consistent with predictions of malaria eradication in the country by 2030.

This will be possible if the country will implement the following recommendations. First, the country should ensure regular monitoring the performance of the Ugandan National Malaria Control Program (UNMCP) to ensure prevention strategies are appropriate. Clinical-based evidence serves as a reliable monitoring tool (Otten, 2009). Secondly, Uganda should enhance the availability of antimalarial drugs, primarily live-saving ACTs to health facilities. This will ensure prompt treatment. Thirdly, the country should develop appropriate strategies to address challenges related to cultural beliefs and practices to promote treatment outcomes.

References

Acton, Q. A. (2012). *Protozoan Infections—Advances in Research and Treatment: 2012 Edition*. Atlanta, GA: Scholarly Editions.

Acton, Q.A (2013). *Parasitic Diseases—Advances in Research and Treatment: 2013 Edition: Scholarly Brief*. Atlanta, GA: Scholarly Editions.

Adams, L. V. & Spielberg, L. A. (2011). *Africa: A Practical Guide for Global Health Workers*. UPNE.

Ahaibwe, G. & Kasirye, I. (2012). Reducing the Burden of Malaria among Children in Uganda. *Economic Policy Research Centre*, 10: 1-4. Retrieved from http://www.eprc.or.ug/pdf_files/policybrief20.pdf

Beaudrap, P. et al. (2011). Heterogeneous Decrease in Malaria Prevalence in Children over a Six-Year Period in South-Western Uganda. *Malaria Journal*, 10:132 doi:10.1186/1475-2875-10-132

Chimp Reports (2013, May 8). Uganda Ranked Highest In Malaria Transmission. *Chimp Media Ltd*. Retrieved from http://chimpreports.com/index.php/people/health/9897-uganda-ranked-highest-in-malaria-transmission.html

Jensen, T. P et al. (2009).Use of the Slide Positivity Rate to Estimate Changes in Malaria Incidence in A Cohort Of Ugandan Children. *Malaria Journal*, 8:213.

Kagolo, F. (2013). *Uganda Improves In Malaria Fight*. Retrieved from http://www.newvision.co.ug/mobile/Detail.aspx?NewsID=630591&CatID=1

Kansiime, D. (2013). *Challenges remain as Uganda achieves the first Millennium Development Goal*. Retrieved from http://www.ug.undp.org/content/uganda/en/home/presscenter/articles/2013/10/17/challenges-remain-as-uganda-achieves-the-first-millennium-development-goal/

Mallinga, S. et al. (2009). *Uganda Malaria Indicator Survey 2009*. Retrieved from http://dhsprogram.com/pubs/pdf/MIS6/MIS6.pdf

Memoire, A. (2011). *Uganda Malaria Programme Performance Review*. Retrieved from http://www.rollbackmalaria.org/countryaction/aideMemoire/Uganda-The-malaria-program-performance-review-2011.pdf

Otten, M. et al. (2009). Initial Evidence of Reduction of Malaria Cases and Deaths in Rwanda and Ethiopia Due To Rapid Scale-Up of Malaria Prevention and Treatment. *Malaria Journal*, 8:14. doi: 10.1186/1475-2875-8-14.

UNICEF (2013). *Uganda: Statistics*. Retrieved from http://www.unicef.org/infobycountry/uganda_statistics.html

Zaramba, S. (2010). *Uganda Malaria Control Strategic Plan 2005/06 – 2009/10*. Retrieved from http://www.rbm.who.int/countryaction/nsp/uganda.pdf

YOUR KNOWLEDGE HAS VALUE

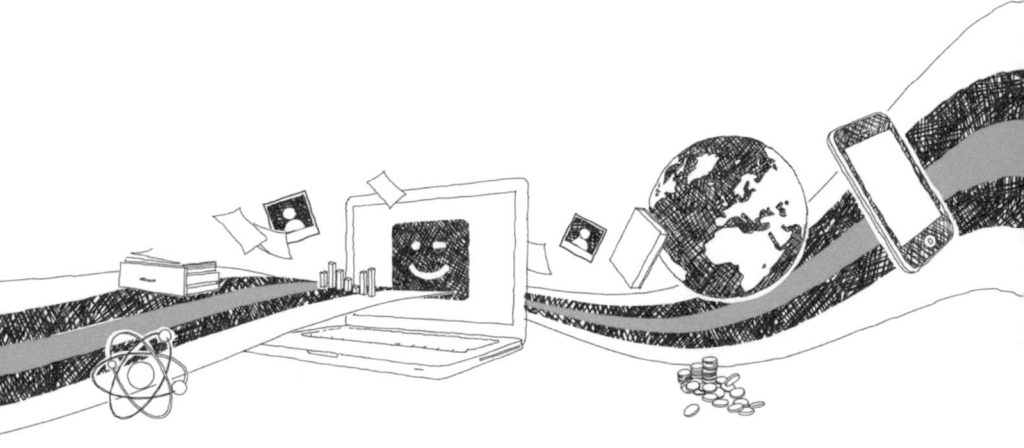

- We will publish your bachelor's and master's thesis, essays and papers

- Your own eBook and book - sold worldwide in all relevant shops

- Earn money with each sale

Upload your text at www.GRIN.com
and publish for free

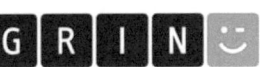